How to train and finish your first 5k race.
By Andreas Michaelides

How to train and finish your first 5k race. Print version

ISBN NUMBER: 978-9963-2209-5-3

CYPRUS LIBRARY

www.cypruslibrary.gov.cy

"There are in fact two things, science, and opinion; the former begets knowledge, the latter ignorance."

— Hippocrates

"Let food be thy medicine and medicine be thy food."

— Hippocrates

"Walking is man's best medicine. "

— Hippocrates

Table of Contents

About The Author.

Andreas was born in Athens, the city that gave birth to Democracy, in Greece, the country that taught to the world how to live, think, and have fun. He grew up in the beautiful island of Cyprus.

With both of his parents bibliophiles (and his father a high school teacher), Andreas grew up with a love and appreciation for literature. In addition to the books he borrowed from the school library, a stack of encyclopedias taught him about the world. A history lover from age 13, he devoured the memoirs of Winston Churchill and Charles de Gaul, and by age 17, he had read all of Julius Vern's books.

After serving his country for 26 months immediately after finishing high school, Andreas studied in Patra, Greece to become a computer engineer. With his Master of Computer Engineering and Informatics, he began working in the Informatics Department of the local university hospital, and started reading again with a vengeance.

In 2004, Andreas authored his first book, a historical novel that has not yet seen the light of publication. Leaving it unpublished made him feel like a failure, but a lot has changed since then. Eleven years later, he has successfully quit smoking and has been smoke-free for the past six years. He has also started running again and managed to lose 26 kg (57 lbs).

Andreas has run three marathons, as well as many half-marathons and other shorter races. His love for running is what renewed him and actually saved his life.

Multiple medical problems pushed Andreas to research and experiment with a plant-based diet; since 2013 he is following a whole plant based diet.

In addition to running, Andreas enjoys hiking, cycling, playing basketball, camping, photography, and going out with friends and family and having a good time.

You can follow the writer at his webpage www.thirsty4health.com and blog http://thirsty4health.com/blog

Why start running anyway?

My intentions of writing this book are honest and they come from the heart.
This book is written for the people who have never practiced the wonderful act of running on a conscious level.
My honest hope is that, with this book, I will inspire people to start running. Running is the only athletic activity that someone could truly say we were born to do (If, of course, we don't have a serious medical condition).

Running is what kept us safe from beasts in the jungle and running is what helped us find food when the vegetation of the planet became scarce and we had to start hunting animals to supplement.
Our brain, this wonderful organ, is still hardwired to tell the body to run whenever there is a need for it.

Why would anyone in their right mind want to start running anyway? I mean, running is very tiring; it actually requires a lot of physical effort, effort that will make you sweaty and often dirty because either you run on dirt roads where you get muddy or you run in a city where you will be breathing all those unhealthy fumes from the cars passing you by on the road every 2 seconds.

Also, the worst part after you finished with all the sweating and trying to avoid being killed by crazy drivers, after your body cools down, it will start aching everywhere feeling like you were hit by a truck. You will feel like your lungs are ready to explode because they cannot handle the sheer quantity of oxygen you need to overcome the physical activity you just did, or feel like someone is reaching into your chest and trying to pull your lungs out.

While your lungs are screaming for air, there is also this awful burning sensation in all of your muscles, which are full of the lactic acid that was created because of the fact that you have been out of shape for years. Your bones also will ache and creak.

Basically, you will feel miserable and in pain and all because you had this bright idea that *running is good for you*. Well, guess again. Why didn't you just stayed home on your comfortable couch, in front of your big screen TV where you can watch your favorite movies while enjoying a few tasty, salty potato chips, washing them down with a cold beer. Oh, yeah, baby, that's the life, right?

Why did you have to leave your favorite chair with the soft pillows and the inviting arms? The chair that wants to serve you and accommodate you while you can have a huge crispy slice of pizza with a double layer of yellow, creamy cheese in one hand and a nice cold soda on the other, watching other people run and sweat for you. Sounds so comfortable and cool, right?

You can watch other people running on the TV, playing football, basketball, or baseball. At least those guys are getting paid to run and jump and tackle. Why should you go through this torture of actually getting up from your soft chair and making yourself go through this ordeal? Why would you enter this nightmare? Why not continue your ignorant bliss of a lovely sedentary life where all you need to do is push the buttons of a remote control and then people in the box can live your desires, your fantasies, your dreams, and ultimately, your life?

Well, people, I'll tell you why.

First Reason: For your Health and Fitness

Yes, it's true my meat, dairy, and processed food eating, sedentary persons. Running is the best exercise to start if you want to be a healthy individual. Running makes your lungs, muscles, and bones stronger; you also get a bigger heart, physically, emotionally, and psychologically.

Running is the sport with the lowest cost. You just get up off your butt, open the front door of your house, and start running in any direction you feel comfortable with at the current moment. You define the pace you want to keep, the distance you want to cover, and the most important of all, you decide if it's going to be fun or not.

You don't even have to run for hours. You only need to exercise the wonderful act of running about 150 minutes per week! That's like 21 minutes every day!

When you start running, you get a lot of benefits. Some of them are prevention of obesity, cardiovascular diseases (heart disease), some forms of cancers, strokes, high blood pressure, type 2 diabetes, and a plethora of other so called chronic illness and diseases of the modern western countries.

If you aren't persuaded to start running just from reading the benefits above, then I have some more for you.

Running makes you a happier individual. When you run, your body releases happy hormones (endocannabinoids), which help you feel better. That's why a lot of doctors today recommend starting a form of exercise to people diagnosed with clinical depression instead of pumping them full of drugs. And running seems to be the best for releasing these nice happy hormones.

Personally, I always feel so much happier and uplifted after a good run and I get what is referred to as a runner high. You need to feel it to understand it; I cannot describe it with words here but you can learn more about my running adventures in my first book, Thirsty for Health.

Also, these wonderful hormones help you cope with anxiety and stress! If that's not a good reason to start running, I don't know what is.

We are talking about natural "drugs" here, people, free from any side effects, ready to flow through your veins at your command. The only thing you need to do is get out there and start running. So still not convinced?

Well, I better continue then.

It makes you look better, because running will help you lose weight and combined with a good diet, preferably a vegetarian one, a vegan diet is even better; you will see that weight around your waist to gradually disappear.

The cool thing about running is that after you stop running, the calorie burning continues well after you finished. How awesome is that? Still not convinced?

Okay, I'll go on then.

Running will help you live longer. When you run, you are gradually making your heart to work more efficiently and in the end, your heart will do the same work load with fewer heart beats.

When I was 92 kilos and a complete couch potato, my heart rate was between 85 to 95 heart beats per minute. Now, after

6 years of running and 20 kilos lighter, my heart rate is 50 to 60 beats per minute; you can learn more about my weight loss struggles in my first book, **Thirsty for Health**.

A good working heart will keep you away from heart diseases and will add years to your life.

I can go on and on about how running will improve your life and make you a happier person but if you don't have the determination to do it, then all of my words here are not going to convince you, because in the end, people, it's you who needs to get up off your comfy chair and start shaping that body into a lean, mean, sexy machine and no one else. If you want to find out how I did it, you can buy my first book, **Thirsty for Health**.

Let me give you another few reasons of why running is all advantages and positives.

1. Overall mental health (Makes you happier as I mentioned)
2. Strengthens your immune system (I have not had a flu for the last six years). By running, you make your immune system stronger, enabling it to fight viruses and bacteria more efficiently.
3. Running increases your learning capabilities and also improves your memory.
4. Another added bonus is that runners can hear better on both low and high frequencies.
5. It helps you sleep better. Any readers suffering from insomnia here?

Second reason: To impress the ladies

If you don't want to start running, I just want to mention a scientifically proven fact that women like fit men. Do you hear that dudes? Women love six packs and broad shoulders and tight gluts. Yes, yes, they do.

To be fair to the fairest of the sexes, they do give more emphasis on the inner world of a man but they also like a man who packs some muscles. They see it as sign of good health and the unconscious of the women makes them to see it as a sign that this male is suitable to be a good partner, a good protector and provider for them.

Trust me, beautiful; hot, gorgeous women do not like couch potatoes with a big belly that are unable to do any physical exercise like walking, running, cycling, going places together, dancing and other more pleasurable activities and poses (wink).

Because my fellow men, beautiful, hot, gorgeous women are usually fit and like to do exercise. Trust me, when I run at racing events, you can see a lot of pretty, hot, sexy women around.

Running is a good way to lose that spare tireyou has around your waist and also improves your health and external appearance.

Also, running makes better partners. Yes, you heard right.

Women perceive running as an important sign of a good breeding partner. Also, regular and consistent running does improve your stamina and I don't just mean in the track ..... If you get my drift.

Thirst reason: To boost your confidence and self esteem.

First, let's see what confidence and esteem means anyway.

Confidence is to have faith in someone or to be able to trust a person or a system.

Now self-confidence basically is to be able to have faith and trust in you.
Esteem is respect and admiration so self-esteem is the ability of a person to respect and admire his or herself.

Some people, everyday people, are so beautiful and even when other people tell them that they are beautiful, they do not believe it because of low confidence and low self-esteem.
Another classic example, which happens a lot in working places and especially in working groups, is in a group of people working on a project, there are using some people who work better, more efficiently, and who produce more than others in the team. Those people are usually the people who do not get the credit and end up staying in the background because they don't want to do the presentation of the project; they don't feel confident enough that they can do it. So people who did not work as hard as the others, but have self-confidence, end up taking the credit.
People do not apply for interviews for a new job because they think they are inadequate or don't fulfill the criteria. Even if they are over-qualified and right for the job, the lack of self-confidence and self-esteem denies and limits their opportunities in every aspect of their life.

Start running and I promise you, every step you make doesn't have to be running at first, just walking; you will transform yourself into a confident person with high self-esteem, full of life and opportunities.

Now let's see how running can boost self-confidence and self-esteem.

If you take running seriously and start to walk/run a certain distance every day, increasing it gradually, then a sense of accomplishment will start to crawl into your mind. Soon, you will realize that you will start to feel invincible; you will feel that there is nothing you cannot do as long you set your goals and manage your time to accomplish it.

Running can do that for you because to be able to finish a race, for example, you need to apply yourself to follow a program. This procedure and the experience you accumulate will make you realize that you can do stuff other than just sitting in front of a TV, being just a daydreamer of what if's. Running will transform you into a doer.

I can't describe the feeling of enormous pride I had when I managed to run my first mile after over 18 years of sedentary life where I abused my body with a range of bad habits and nutrition mistakes. If you want to learn more about of how I managed to overcome my addictions, you can buy my first book, **Thirsty for Health**.

In a nutshell, running can improve your self-confidence by making you:

Feel better and stronger, and look better. It gives you a sense of accomplishment, reduces stress, and actually alters the physiology of your brain, making you smarter! Also, by setting a plan and achieving your goals through a well thought out program, you can help give yourself a greater sense of empowerment that will leave you feeling much happier and in the end, much healthier.

To socialize and make friends

I have read a lot of books about running and there is this agreement that running is a primarily a lonely athletic endeavor. There is some truth in that. When I started running 6 years ago, it was fine to run alone at first. I loved the fact that was no one around to make fun of the little fat boy running around the high school track like a hamster in his little wheel. I liked it because I didn't have to explain to people why I run and I also wanted to avoid contact with people that consider running as a waste of time, like many of you think right now reading this book.

Well, guess what? You are not going to find any people criticizing running on a running track, on a scenic dirt road, or a nice seaside running trail, who consider running as a waste of time. You will only find individuals who consider running an advantage that gives you all those wonderful benefits I described already in this book.

After I lost my first kilos in the first six months (walking in the beginning, a transition period of walking/running, and finally, purely running), my self-confidence and self-esteem skyrocketed. For a while, I felt invincible and for the first time, in control of my life.
After that initial boost of self-confidence and self-esteem that running provided me, I started to consider why I run now that I lost the weight.
I had that feeling of emptiness when I was running. I need to admit, as I already mention in my first book, **Thirsty for Health**, my motivation for running was driven from pure vanity. I didn't like the way I looked so I started running to lose weight and after I achieved that, I would stop.
Down the road, though, I discovered all the wonderful benefits of running and I did not stop.

What helped me keep running and helped me learn more about nutrition and other important and interesting topics was that running gave me the opportunity to meet new people and make friends. People who had similar stories and interests such as running helped me reach another level of enlightenment.

I met a lot of people through running. Some of them, I became friends with and with others; I exchange stories and information about running and nutrition. It gave me a sense that I belonged to a rare kind of group, now the runners group, a new tribe I entered and I passed my initiation with flying colors. You can be part of this wonderful tribe called runners. All you have to do is get up off your couch, find a running buddy, if you wish, and start running.
You can support each other; don't let each other quit the effort.
The best thing you can do is find a running club near you and start running with them. Runners are very polite people and we love helping newbie's. You have more chances of starting running and incorporating into your life than alone, I am not saying that you will not be able to do it alone, but statistics show that if you are in a group with similar mindset and intentions, you have more possibilities to succeed.

To lose weight.

Most people, when they start running, including me, started with the intention of losing weight. They woke up one morning, saw themselves in their bathroom or bedroom mirror, and for the first time in their life, in years, saw their real physique. They saw a fat person looking back at them, a complete stranger; someone had invaded in their mirror and was looking back at them.
That's not possible, that can't be me. Who is that fat man looking back at me with their belly sticking out like a balloon?

That's not me. No, no. Who is that fat woman looking back at me with the saggy breasts, full moon face, and loose and relaxed behind?

Most of us, like I mention in my first book, **Thirsty for Health**, when we see ourselves in the mirror, we don't see the reality but a version of the reality they want to see. Our brain, this amazing organ, can project the image we desire and make us see that image as real. This condition is called living in denial.

My exhortation to you is that starting to run to lose weight is an amazing way, an excellent way, to lose weight quick; losing weight will make you faster and healthier. My advice, though, is this: do not base your hopes only on running to lose the extra fat. You need to combine it with a healthy dietary and nutritional lifestyle. Pay attention to what I said, I said lifestyle, not diet. You need to start running and stick with it and also adopt a plant-based diet preferably to see healthy and permanent results.

It's not rocket science, people, is plain math; it's calories in and calories out. If you eat more calories than your body needs, you gain weight. If you eat less calories than you need, you will lose weight.

If you start running without following a healthy nutritional regime and lifestyle, then you will not lose any fat and you will end up quitting because of the poor results you will have.

That's was my two cents' worth of losing weight through the lovely exercise of running.

Plus, for every pound you lose, you become two seconds faster per mile. The secret is to maintain the same number of calories you consume and increase the level of exercise, which will allow you to burn more calories than you eat.

You can make a free account on a various dietary tracking sites(my favorite is www.cronometer.com).You can record what you eat everyday and what kind of exercise you do, and you can set your goal there and it will show you how many calories you consume and how many burned. Of course, these sites do not give you the exact calories that went in and out but they give you an estimation.

Trust me, in time, you will be so knowledgeable of what goes into your mouth, you will not even need the online calorie tracker.

Unknown (To see what will happen)

People are, by nature, afraid of the unknown; I used to be like those people. But once I I realized that you can conquer the unknown through systematic, persistent search and research.I stopped being afraid and a sense of freedom took over me. It's like I mention in one of my articles, "The Power of Knowledge", posted on my webpage.

There is a simple formula you can follow to conquer the unknown, which is:

1. Research
2. Experiment
3. Apply
4. Conclude
5. Correct your mistakes
6. Repeat!

Now what I fear the most is not the unknown but is ignorant people who think they know everything.

Stop being ignorant, killing yourself with every bite of processed food and dead flesh, dairy, and other products that were produced through pain and agony (the slaughter of the animal kingdom so we can have a steak Saturday night).

Break the ignorance, start running, and I promise you, the veil of not knowing will be lifted; the fog in your mind of why the world is like this will be dissolved.

Do a medical checkup.

As long as I live, I will never forget the day I started walking, which eventually turned into running. It was 26 of April 2010; it was around 8 p.m. night at the high school track of my village.

I had stopped smoking about a year before, so it was only natural that I gained a lot of kilos as a lot of ex-smokers know. There I was, a fat dude standing at the start of the hundred meter startup line, looking down the track, wondering how the heck I managed to be 92 kilos at the age of 35.

As I describe in my first book, Thirsty for Health, I did walk 3 loops that night and that was the beginning of a beautiful journey that is still in progress and will end when I die and I hope with my new found and adopted lifestyle, plant-based nutrition, to be at least 100 years old. Well, unless a bus runs me over (wink).

My mistake was that I did not do a cardiograph; I was one of the lucky people who had, and still has, a good working heart.
With all the meat, fish, and dairy I consumed the previous years, the lack of exercise for 11 years, it did mess up my health and had serious complications in other organs of my body like having stomach and duodenum ulcer, esophageal ulcer, constipation hemorrhoids, heartburn, migraines, and so many other illness and diseases; you can read all about it in my first book, Thirsty for Health.
I was lucky my heart was in good shape when I started running, I can't even imagine the thought of something being wrong with the "old ticker" and I would start running and ending up having a heart attack or, even worse, dying.
My advice is before you start exercising, not just for running; take a cardiograph and also some blood general exams, electrolytes exams, and your thyroid.

After you do that, take the results, go to a doctor, tell him/her that you want to start exercising and the type of exercise you want to do, and only start running if you get the okay from the doc. don't be a fool like I was, be smart.

Of course, you can do the opposite, go to your doctor tell him/her what your intentions are towards starting an exercise regime and he/she will tell you what kind of tests to take.

Now, every time I start my training period, I always go and do a cardiograph, and, of course, the other exams I mentioned at least once a year.

Set your Goal.

If you have decided to get rid your sedentary past, if you have really taken it upon yourself to change the way your life is and where it is heading, then setting your goal is maybe the most important factor to allow you to be successful on your endeavor of running. With wisdom, prudence, and deep thinking, nothing is impossible.

From my experience of running the last 6 years and the mistakes I made, setting your goal falls into the next three steps, and must be followed in order.

- *Just finish, time is not an issue*

If you are a newbie and have never run before in your life, then this is your best goal: just finish the race. You will be able to walk/run with no time to constrain you and stress you out. My advice from personal experience, and also from other people I talk with, your first 5k race should be as carefree as possible. This will enable you to have fun. That's why most of the 5k races the organizers christen them fun run, fun race, and it will make you love running even more and not end up hating it because you set goals that you could not fulfill in the first place. Try and find a 5k race that does not have a time limit or one that is in a safe area like a park and not on a public street. This way, you won't have to worry about cars coming at you after the time limit has ended and certain roads are returned back to traffic.

Finish in the boundaries of the race organizers

All the races have time boundaries on the race. This is done for various reasons. Sometimes, races close traffic down and it's important to return the roads to the traffic as soon as possible, and another reason is that it will ensure that records will be made if you keep the time limit of the race short, like Boston Marathon is. For every age group, you have to achieve a minimum time in previous marathons to be able to participate in the race. This makes the race more difficult and gives it more prestige.
This goal, and I am always talking from experience, talking with other runners, and, of course, from a lot of books I have read about running, this kind of goal should be set after you done a couple of stress-free 5k fun races. You have seen how it is done, you went over the initial fears and anxieties you may had about the race, and now you are ready to challenge yourself to another level.

Run like the devil is on your tail

This goal is a goal that must be set after you did some 5ks and manage to finish them below the cut off time of the race. By now, you are not a recreational person who runs for fun. You are at the first levels of becoming a runner and starting to challenge yourself to see if you can finish that next 5k faster than the previous. Trust me, if you stick with running, the competitive bug will kick in and the only thing you can do to deal with it is to go with it and embrace it. That's what I did when I started running half-marathons, as I describe in my first book, **Thirsty for Health**.

Alone or with Company

I did touch on this issue briefly when I was talking about socializing and making friends. Yes, it's true, running will take you to roads you never thought you will follow and situations you never dreamed would happen to you.

You will meet crazy people, sane people, elite athletes, recreational athletes, people running with their kids, grandparents running with their grandkids. The tribe of runners has a lot of peculiarities and a lot of colors, both of the uniforms they wear and the color of their skin. You will see black, white, dark colored, Asian, mixed races, and so on, but they all have one thing in common. When they all come together to a starting line, ready to begin, in their faces, you can see this incredible pride and satisfaction that they managed to find the time and put in the effort to train for this 5k or any other distance race.

Now the question is run with a friend a group of people, like a running club, or alone. Well, for me, it was the third choice. Before I met my wife, I would run and train alone, something that sometimes was cool but sometimes, I would have these really intense lonely moments where I wish someone else was there with me training, supporting me, and helping me, and I would have done the same. Runners are people who help each other and we have this unbelievable sense of altruism and sacrifice for our fellow runners.

Even if you are selfish, after you start running, you will see a dramatic change into you and that is you will become healthier, happier, nicer, and more compassionate to other people and to yourself.

I remember my ex-wife when she had her first 5k and you should have seen her face when she got her finisher medal, all red from the effort, of course, but full of pride and unbelievable satisfaction. Of course, the next few days, she was all sore in her legs but no pain, no gain, as they say.

So if you ask me what is best, alone, with a friend, or with a group of people, my answer is that you need to try three options and then make a wise decision. You never know if the friend you find to train with will go all the way or give up, taking you with him/her. That's a disadvantage and advantage of training with a friend. You will help each other mentally and psychologically, making sure you will not quit. A good thing to do is to find a friend who is already a runner and is willing to help you with everything you need to know because you are a newbie and all.

In the situation where you don't want to train alone either because you don't know how or your self-esteem and self-confidence is down, then I suggest finding a running club in your area and go join it. It's the perfect and ideal situation for a newbie because you will meet other newbies, too, so you won't feel alone. Also, the older runners will help you with everything you need, and help you to keep it up and not quit.

Gear up

Besides being one of the best ways to boost your immune system resulting in a better healthier version of you, running is maybe the easiest and economic athletic activity out there.
All you need is decent running shoes, some shorts, a t-shirt, and a hat, but let's take a look at them briefly one by one.

Clothes

A running t-shirt, running shorts, socks, and a hat is all you need to start exercising and applying the wonderful athletic activity of putting one leg in front of the other in a rhythmic steady pace.

Your clothes will depend heavily on the seasonal changes and variations of where you train and also where you will race. It's a good tactic to simulate your training in weather conditions similar to that of the place where the race will be held. I mean, you will never train in a hot climate and go race in a cold climate and vice versa it just don't make any sense, plus if you do that you will not achieve the goals you set up.

In a nutshell

When the weather is neutral to hot, you want to wear less and loose clothing so your body will be able to get rid of all the heat that is generated through your running effort.

When the weather is high in humidity, your best bet is to keep less and loose clothing but in addition, drink lots of fluids, water, and electrolytes and also slow your pace, unless you want to be covered in sweat in the first mile of your run. High humidity weather, for me, is my nightmare. I sweat a lot now, imagine all that humidity blocking my sweat from evaporating into the air. Yep, I am literally swimming in my sweat from the first mile.

When the weather is cold, well, this is a no brainer. When you are going to run in a cold weather environment, you should think about onion. Yes, you heard me right, think of onion. What does an onion have? Well, it has lots and lots of layers.
When you run in freezing conditions, you need to ensure that heat does not escape your body; otherwise you will have your little tushy frozen in a matter of minutes so the secret is to wear multiple layers of clothing that will trap the air between them. Trapped air is one of the best materials to achieve insulation.

The inner material that touches your skin should be polypropylene so moisture is carried away from the skin.

When there is wind and rain while you train, you need to make sure your outer layer of clothing is water and wind resistant (doh) (smile)

Experiment with your clothes and you will figure out what best suits you. Every person is unique as I say many times in my first book, Thirsty for Health.

A few tips more about two situations you are going to encounter.

One is the so called running nipples. If you decide to take this 5k challenge, and I am sure you will get hooked as I was, then you are going to want to run further and faster. You mark my words, after a few 5ks, your body and the new version of you will ache to try a 10k race or even a 21k race. When you start doing that, you will inevitably run longer and the longer you run, then chances are, you will get bloody nipples. Yes, you heard me right. This applies for both sexes, men and women.

I remember I would go take a shower after I did my first a 16k training session and to my surprise, I noticed that both of my nipples were bleeding. The right one was worse. Calm down, I wasn't bleeding to death but they sure were painful to say the least.

Me not knowing what it was, I assumed the worst, like something was wrong with me. It was after a few more 16k training races and a few more bleeding nipples that I made the connection and researched it even more, dusting off my running books, and found out that it was caused by the friction of my ill-suited t-shirt and my sweat.

There are a few preventive solutions you can apply; trust me, you do not want this on your hands, or in this case, on your chest (wink).

You can cover them with Band-Aids. I tried that but it did not work for me after a while because of the sweat. Yes, I am a sweater. They come off, so that did not work for me.

What I found really efficient and economic is applying of Vaseline on my nipples. If you find an organic substitute of Vaseline, even better, because let's face it, people, Vaseline is a petroleum product, and the last thing I want is petrol on my skin.

I used Vaseline for many years, it did the work of protecting my nipples from the friction but at what cost? At the same time, I was injecting myself with chemicals through my skin.

It was my ex-wife, who opened my eyes and made me see that petroleum-based Vaseline is not good for me. Now I use an organic, handmade ointment made out of thyme and wax and It works like Vaseline, plus, it smells awesome.

A third way, a bit more expensive, is to invest in a couple of special t-shirts (for women, a good running bra) that transport the sweat to the outside layer and cannot become saturated with moisture.

For someone who just starts running and just wants to finish a couple of 5k before moving on to longer races, this is not an issue. An issue for you newbies, especially if you are overweight, is the next problem, which is called chaffing, often of the skin on the inner thighs.

Now that happens because your exposed, fatty thighs are rubbing together. Applying a good portion of Vaseline, organic or not, is your call, but you can always wear longer shorts.

Shoes

Now you can get away with some simple trainers at the start of your training but if you really want to incorporate running into your life, making it a lifestyle, then you will need to invest in the future in the acquisition of a good pair of running shoes.

To be honest, to this day, after 6 years of running, I don't know as much as I would like to know about shoes. I know enough but I feel I need to learn a little bit more to be able to better improve my running speed and performance.

When I am shopping for running shoes, I make sure to wear them at least 10 minutes, walking up and down to see how they feel and I always wear, or bring, the socks I will be training in to see how that shoe is on my feet.

You don't want to buy a shoe that is too small or too big. You need to pay extra attention so the shoe feels comfortable on you.

Always shop for shoes, including running shoes, in the morning rather than in the afternoon because feet swell during the day. Also, always leave some space for the toes, especially the big toe. As you run, the big toe gets bigger because of the swelling; plus, keep in mind that your feet are not exactly the same size so always make sure you are comfortable with the bigger foot.

If you don't feel that you can make it on your own, you can always ask for the help of a specialist, like a podiatrist (foot doctor) to diagnose what kind of feet you have. Also, you can always go and shop for your shoes from stores that employ professionals who will help you with picking the right shoe for you. Another bit of advice is if you find a good pair of running shoes that are perfect for you, stock up. If you think that you can find it 6 months from now, then you are mistaken. I always buy two pairs of shoes that I find perfect for me and I never regret it.

So, come on, start using the Internet, search for some good sport stores in your neighborhood and start taking your life back!

In closing, when you wear your running shoe, it should feel like an extension of your foot, not like strange part glued on your feet.

Where and when to train?

That's an interesting question. In this hectic lifestyle we all live, sometimes finding a little bit of time just to do something for us looks impossible. Especially so if you are married and even worse when you have a bunch of little images of you running around, bringing havoc and chaos to your life, crying, not letting you sleep, and all the other wonderful activities of parenting. (smile)

Well, my advice is simple. Pull yourself together, use that brain of yours and sit down and make a schedule, a realistic one, and stick with it.

Once you go through it, note any mistakes you make or things you can improve or things you want to remove and so on. The next time, make a better schedule and you be more efficient with both your running and your family.

Try to incorporate and convince family members to join you on your running training sessions, not at first but gradually.

Now if you are single, then you have no reason for not going for a running training at least 4 times a week. It doesn't have to be every day; plus, running everyday is not good for you. I personally have two days off from running a week. I train and run the other five, which gives me the opportunity to get some rest and also recharge my love for running.

If you are single, you can do your training sessions in the morning before you go to work. That applies for married people, too! You can get up when everyone is sleeping, go do your thing, and come back as if nothing happened. Another thing is that if you can't do that because you have little babies crying, you can ask your partner to take care of them while you can have your morning run. If he/she loves you, he/she will do it for you.

You see where I am going with this. The day has 24 hours, clear your mind and I am sure you will be able to find an hour to do your running sessions. Actually, in the beginning, only 15 to 30 minutes will be enough, at least 4 times a week, as you get more into shape, and then you can figure it out where to find the extra time. And trust me, those 15 to 20 minutes every time you go for a run or a training session will be the most productive minutes of your day.

While you walk or run, solutions to everyday problems will pop into your head and you will speak and mumble to yourself questions like "Why on earth I didn't think of that before?"Or "Wow, that was so obvious, where was my mind all this time?"

Well, let me tell you something, and I have really researched this, when you run, your brain creates new neural pathways, which means, people, that with running, we are becoming smarter! Literally smarter!

If you are unemployed, then what's your excuse? You can run any time of the day.

If you can't go run in the morning, then see if you can go after work or later into the day. Just find the time, make the time, schedule, program yourself, put your thinking cap on, and **JUST MAKE TIME FOR YOU!**

When I started running 6 years ago, I had 3 jobs. Yes, that's right, you heard me right, 3 jobs, I would go to sleep at midnight, wake up 5 a.m. the next day, and work until midnight again, and so on and so on.

I was making good money, I wasn't a millionaire but I wasn't starving, I was doing okay. So what I thought, in those 5 years of doing this, I had chronic constipation. Almost every day, I was hit by hemorrhoids, heartburn, stomach upsets, I was fat and had trouble breathing, my blood pressure was flirting with hypertension, and I was only 35 years old!

So one night, after I saw myself in the mirror, and as I already mentioned earlier in this book, *saw* myself as I really was for the first time, I just got into my car drove to the nearest high school track and ran 3 loops before I stopped because I couldn't breathe anymore. In that moment, a zillion thoughts passed through my mind as I describe in my first book (in the Running chapter), Thirsty for Health, available both in Kindle and Paperback edition.

After that awakening and that first "run", I scheduled walking at first and then running two times a day. I would go walk for 30 minutes after I was done with my morning job and then another 30 minutes after I was done with my afternoon job.

I had three jobs, people, and I managed to walk an hour every day. I am sure *YOU* can do the same; I don't want to hear any excuses *JUST DO IT!*

Now, where to train. It all depends on where you live. A lot of people I know, especially those living in the city, they just gear up and they start running from their front door, do a nice loop, and come back.

Others go by car or by bike to a park and do their training or to a high school track to do their training there. I am sure, wherever you are; you will find a place to train.

Other don't even have to leave their house. They invested in a treadmill and they transformed themselves from couch potatoes watching TV to treadmill potatoes watching TV (smile).The possibilities are endless. The only thing confining you is your mind, so let your mind expand and set it free and running, I am sure, will help you do that. It will help your mindset, too, besides doing wonders for your health and your fitness level.

On your own or Hire a Pro

This is a personal choice and personally, I always loved, and still love, to find out stuff on my own. I consider it to be more important for me to find the information that will shape me into the image I have in my mind. I give you an example. For many years since I started running, I considered warming up and cooling down exercises a waste of time. You know, you go to a race, everyone is running up and down like crazy, stretching everywhere, and there was me just standing there, looking at all those "clowns" wasting energy.

Well, guess what? The "clown" was me! After having a few injuries that could have been easily avoided if I did as little as 5 minutes of warm-up and 10 minutes of cool down sessions, I learned the importance of warming up and cooling down.

Now a religious fanatic of yoga, warming up, cool down, and rehabilitation exercises, I have a day just for relaxing and stretching yoga-like exercises.

Anyway, if you go alone, you are going to have your ups and downs and hopefully, you will learn from your mistakes. If you feel that you don't want to do the research on your own, either you don't have the time or any other reason, you can seek the help of a trained professional; there is no shame in that.

That's my two cents on the matter.

Diet and Nutrition

This will be a work in progress for you because every person is a different, unique, and special entity on this wonderful planet of ours.

I am going to tell you a few things about me. Most of them are already mentioned in my first book, **Thirsty for Health**.

When I started running almost six years ago, I was an omnivore, meaning I would eat anything. It was the beginning of my journey and the reason I started running in the first place was vanity. I was using running as a tool to shed those extra kilos and then I would stop.
That was the initial plan anyway, to make a long story short, here I am writing a free book on how to train and finish your first 5k, trying to convince potato people like you to start running.

I was a couch potato; a big one. I would sit in front of my computer screen with my snacks, dips and chips and sodas and popcorn full of salt, and I would watch movie after movie and at the same time, I would eat that yummy(what I thought) junk food nonstop.

Other times, I would be playing an online strategy game for hours, eating and drinking junk food.

Six years later, diet wise, I am a vegan, and have been for the last three years now and I feel great. I am not telling you need to become a strict vegetarian like me to be able to run a 5k race but maybe after you lose all that weight and that last 2.5 to 5 pounds left and they refuse to go away, maybe you should look into vegetarian lifestyle.

It is a known fact and a scientific truth that a vegetarian diet will boost your immune system, and improve your running performance.

Make sure you don't eat much food high in cholesterol and saturated fat. Increase your servings of fruits and vegetables. Also increase your water intake, look into electrolytes.

Consult a doctor and a dietician about your future endeavor on starting to run. He or she will tell you what to eat; if you can find a vegan or vegetarian doctor and dietician, even better.

My diet now consists of fruits in the morning, as much as I can eat, then when I come home, I have a big juice made out from carrots and beets, then after about 45 minutes, which how much it usually need for my juice to get digested, I go train with my wife. At the time of writing this, I am training for a 12k trail run in the mountains and my wife is training for a 4k trail running, too.

Then we come home and we usually have some kind of legumes (lentils, beans, chickpeas, peas, black eyes-peas, fava beans) or starch-based food (potatoes, sweet potatoes, brown rice) and we always have a salad on the table, usually a rainbow salad, we try to have all the colors in there.

At night, we usually have our tea and if we get really hungry, we might have a smoothie, or a whole wheat spaghetti or some boiled veggies (broccoli, cauliflower, romanesco).

The secret is to try different foods and see what works for you. Remember, *you are unique!*

This Book goal.

This book goal should be your goal, too, and it is to make you get up from the lounge chair of yours, get your health and your life back, and boost your self-confidence and self-esteem by finishing a 5k race.

It only takes that first step and you make it, I have faith in you, I honestly do because I know how you feel. I was you 6 years ago and I understand and want you to know that you are not alone in this struggle. I will be here helping you with my books and mark my words, you will see that you will meet other people with similar issues and problems as yours and you will relate and connect and you will help each other to attain the unattainable and that is *you* getting off that arm chair and starting to shape your health, your body, and your emotional situation into a better version of your current state.

I am assuming that you are not a couch potato anymore, both in your mind and in reality, I am assuming you have had all your medical checks and the doctor has cleared you for running and for the last few weeks, you have being walking/running for about 30 minutes 3 to 5 times a week.

If you are in that level, then I have a surprise for you! You are ready to start training for your 5k race.

As I said before in this book, and I say it a lot in my first book, **Thirsty for Health**, too, every person is unique. We are snowflakes in beautiful winter scenery in the middle of a frozen lake.

Having said that, my advice is to just finish your first 5k race, let yourself experience it, do not race it, you will have plenty opportunities to race, not just 5k but longer distances like 10k, half-marathon, and even a marathon! No one knows how this will end up, but know this, you are the driver of your life, not society, not anyone else, *you* and only *you*!

So if you set your mind to doing a 5k race, then the following information is for those people who just want to finish their first 5k and not race it. I want to be clear on this.

I am going to write a book on how to race a 5k in the future because I am sure lots of you will want to read that but for the time being, let's focus on the having fun and just finishing part.

Pre-Register

It's a good tactic to register for the race a few months before the event, even if a lot of the races offer race day registration. You don't really want to run at the last minute, waiting on line and plus the fee will be more expensive. So pre-register and have your mind at ease.

Training for your first 5k race.

In the future, you will hear other more experienced runners talking about warming up and cooling down exercises, about speed work, hill work, tempo pace, track repeats, long, short, and mediums runs, strength exercises, and so on. I have good news for you, for this training session, you don't need to worry about these things.

As I said earlier on this book, get a medical checkup, get cleared by a doctor, and let's start training for our 5k race.

A training schedule.

The first thing you need to do is write down a training program that you will follow to the letter as much as you can. The important thing is for the program to be flexible because let's face it, life is life, and events that are not under our control can happen.

For example, let's say you have program to do 2 miles on Friday and you have Saturday off, no running at all, and let's say something happens on Friday and you end up missing doing your 2 miles. Don't worry, consider Friday a day off and do them on Saturday. This is the philosophy behind of a flexible program.

Just because you wrote I need to do something on a specific day doesn't mean it is written in stone so use your heads, people, and be flexible when you are designing your running program.

Keep a running Diary/log

A very good idea and one that I found to be really helpful as far as memory lane is concerned is to keep a running log. My running log really helped me write a big chunk of my first book, Thirsty for Health.

A running log will be your companion and your friend. In times of desperation, in times that you feel you had enough, or in times that you start doubting why you even bother with running, and you are at the verge of quitting, you can read your running log and see how much progress you made, from being a couch potato to a runner, how much weight you lost, how good it makes you feel after you got into your routine.

Write whatever you feel in your running diary, write how fast you run, how much you run, how you feel before, during, and after the race, write about the weather, and write if you had any injuries or pains. This information will help you become a better runner in the future and also a better person; the lessons you will acquire from practicing the sacred art of running will help you in other areas of your life, like your work place, with your family, and with your social circle. The possibilities are endless.

Training Tips

Your weekly distance covered in a week should be at least two to three times the distance of your programmed race. In our case, our race is 5 km so our weekly distance should be between 10 and 15 km.

You should increase your weekly distance by a factor of 10%.For example, if you run 10 km the previous week, next week, you should run 10km plus 10% of 10, which is 1km, so this week, you should run 11km. It's a good rule because it gives the body time to cope with the added stress and do the necessary repairs with safety and ease.

You should have at least 2 days off from running, and those two days away will recharge your batteries and make you achieve better performance; a rest day is as important as a training day.

There are other tips but for those who only wish to finish, those tips do not apply.

Sample 5k training program in miles – Eight weeks – For your first 5k

W.	Mon	Tues	Wed.	Thurs.	Fri.	Sat.	Sun.	Total
1	Off	2m	2m	2m	Off	2m	Off	8
2	Off	2m	2m	2m	Off	2m	2m	10
3	Off	2m	2m	2m	Off	2m	2m	10
4	Off	2m	3m	2m	Off	2m	3m	12
5	Off	2m	3m	2m	Off	2m	3m	12
6	Off	2m	3m	2m	Off	2m	3m	12
7	Off	2m	3m	2m	Off	2m	3m	12
8	Off	2m	2m	2m	Off	2m	Race	8 + 3.1

The days off do not have to be Monday and Friday, you can reshape this program to suit your needs, the important thing is to cover the weekly miles.

It doesn't matter if you do the miles in the morning, in afternoon, or later at night.

Warm up and cooling down.

I want to say a few words about these two very important parts of running. I learned it the hard way that is very important to warm up before starting a training session and cooling down after you finish.

34

Our muscles and tendons are like a well oiled machine and you need to treat them with respect and love.

They take some time to warm up before you should start asking them to go to work. Warming up is like some people's morning coffee; they need to have it to be able to function. Well, warming up exercises are like that, they prepare your body.

I always like to do the least effort and get the best results so this is how I warm up.
I walk for 10 to 15 minutes, it doesn't matter if I am on a track or outside in a trail, I walk for 10 to 15 minutes with a comfortable pace, not too slow but not power walking either.

After that, I will start running for about 10 minutes with a comfortable pace again and after that, I do this.

I start butt kicking myself for about 20 meters and then I run, I stride for about 80 meters, and then I slow down.

On the way back, I do high knee lifts for 20 meters stride for about 80 meters and then slow down, I do that as many times as I feel are necessary.

After that, I start doing what I have planned for the day.

After the training session is over, my cooling down method is pretty simple. I walk for about 10 to 15 minutes until my heart rate drops back to normal.

A few tips about Race day.

If you can go to collect your number and other accessories a day before the race, that would be better and it will remove some of the stress of you running to go get them the day of the race.

Use the shoes and clothes you have been training with. Do not, *I repeat*, do not use new shoes or gear that you did not practice with on race day because that will be a big mistake especially on the feet. I say this especially to women who always want to wear something nice and new to the race. Ladies, it's a 5k race, not a beauty contest.

The other day, my wife almost made the mistake of breaking a new pair of shoes because they were prettier than the ones she used to train for her first 5k. If I hadn't noticed it in time, she would be whining to *me* how her feet hurt. So, people, do not wear anything new on race day; go run with the shoes and gear you trained for so many weeks.

As I said at the beginning of the book, because this is going to be your first race try, find a race near you, and if you find one in walking distance would be ideal.

If you didn't manage to do that and you are not nearby, then you should check out and make sure you know the following information:

- Means of transportation and routes from where you live to the race location
- Parking facilities
- How long it will take you to go there
- Weather conditions so you know what kind of clothes to pack
- Double check the time that the race starts
- Make sure you use the toilet before you head out. Runners get nervous before the event, thus the lines

outside the portable toilets in race locations are not a strange phenomenon.

Once on the site of the race, make sure you do a good warm up like I described earlier. At the starting line, please position yourself at the back or near the back so you will not get sandwiched or run over by speedsters or get dragged into a fast pace. Remember, you there to have fun, not end up in the hospital!

When the race gun goes boom! Start walking, giving the faster runners the opportunity to get out of your way and then start running your routine pace, the one that you practiced during training.
Stick with that and I am sure you will be finishing your first 5k race in no time! Remember to stop and walk while you drink your water from the aids station, be nice to the volunteers and fellow runners and when you are finishing, have a big smile on your face because you deserve it!

Aftermath

After the race, take it easy for a few days. Be lazy, you deserve it. Show your medal to your friends and family, even co-workers, and let them admire you for your achievement. There is nothing to be ashamed of; you have everything to be proud about yourself.

Sit down and write in your diary how you felt before, during, and after the race. Analyze the race, learn from your mistakes, and improve so next time, you'll be better at it.

Congratulations, you are now officially a runner!

Other books by Andreas Michaelides

42 Tips That Will Make You A Better Runner

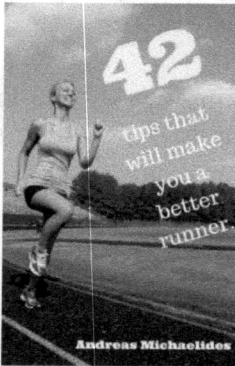

There are of course more than 42 tips that someone can utilize to become a better runner. The reason I chose 42 is entirely personal; they are not the best 42 tips or the most important; they are simply my 42 tips. These are the first 42 tips that popped into my head while I was thinking of what makes a better runner taken out of 6 years of running, from 5km to 50km, and they are also the result of a lot of running injuries and applied knowledge accumulated from other runners and books.

How To Train And Finish Your First 10k Race.

You need to know the theory behind it, the mindset. Second, you need to know the practical aspect of the theory, and last but not least, you need to know the step by step configuration your mind has to follow to achieve that task. Any lack of information in either of the above situations and your rate of success diminishes, and this applies to all the tasks that people set their minds to conquer. I am telling you all these, so you see that the information you are

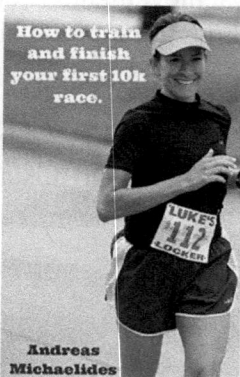

going to read in this book will help you train and finish your first 10km race.

Please write a review.

I consider myself as a person that wants to think that I am constantly improving my books, my work and myself. I am always trying to deliver to my readers the best quality and current information out there as my area of interest and expertise is concern which is Health, Nutrition and Exercise.

In order to accomplish that I need feedback from you and the only feedback I know that will help me achieve a relative perfection in all areas of my life is your valuable reviews so I know where I am wrong or where I have made mistakes and errors.

There is no such thing as a perfect book out there, perfection for one person is a sloppy work for other, so in order to satisfy as much as people out there my books need to be updated regularly and it doesn't matter if its in electronic form (kindle) or paperback form.

If you found this book useful, please leave your review with all your thoughts, don't hold back, it will only take a few minutes of your time.

If you didn't like this book, please let me know by contacting me and I will give my best shot to fix the issue.

Thank you very much,
Andreas

Sources

Books

Galloway's book on running 2nd edition by Jeff Galloway
Chi Running by Danny Dreyer and Katherine Dreyer
The runner's body by Ross Tucker PhD, Jonathan Dugas
PhD, and Mark Fitzgerald
Complete book of Running edited by Amby Burfoot
The runner's handbook by Bob Glover, Jack Shepherd and
Shelly-lynn Florence Glover
Thrive Fitness by Brendan Brazier
Pose method of running by Nicholas Romanov PhD with
John Robson
The non-runner's marathon trainer by David A. Whitsett,
Forrest A. Dolgener and Tanjala Mabon Kole
The competitive runner's handbook by Bob Glover and
Shelly-lynn Florence Glover
Running the Lydiard way by Arthur Lydiard with Garth
Gilmour
Run less run faster by Bill Pierce, Scott Murr and Ray Moss
Run faster from the 5k to the marathon by Brad Hudson and
Matt Fitzrerald

Links

Strength Weights

http://www.runnersworld.com/general-interest/strength-
workouts-may-yield-significant-improvement-in-5k-times
http://www.scienceofrunning.com/2010/05/more-on-
strength-training-for-runners.html
http://www.fitnessmagazine.com/workout/running/5k/5k-
10k-half-marathon-training-plans/

http://www.marathon-training-guides.com/strength-training.html
http://www.moneycrashers.com/weighted-body-bar-exercises/
http://greatist.com/move/lunge-variations-you-need-to-know
http://www.marathon-training-guides.com/strength-exercises.html
http://www.bodybuilding.com/fun/a-new-breed-of-athlete-be-a-strength-runner.html
http://www.flotrack.org/article/21661-to-make-it-to-the-next-level-strength-training-is-a-must

Self Confidence and Self Esteem articles

http://www.empowerthedream.com/boost-esteem-running/
http://zenhabits.net/25-killer-actions-to-boost-your-self-confidence/
http://www.livestrong.com/article/438937-how-does-exercise-affect-your-self-esteem/
http://www.huffingtonpost.com/therese-borchard/sports-self-esteem_b_861317.html
http://www.dailymile.com/blog/uncategorized/developing-self-confidence-through-running-how-i-found-myself-out-on-the-road
http://www.mightyfighter.com/improve-your-self-confidence-and-self-esteem/
http://www.goal-setting-guide.com/ways-exercise-improve-self-confidence/

Health benefits of running

http://www.runnersworld.com/start-running/6-ways-running-improves-your-health
http://runhaven.com/2015/04/06/10-benefits-running-never-knew/
http://www.active.com/running/articles/6-benefits-of-running

http://www.telegraph.co.uk/men/active/11524491/The-surprising-health-benefits-of-going-for-a-run.html
http://greatist.com/fitness/30-convincing-reasons-start-running-now
http://www.shape.com/fitness/cardio/you-dont-have-run-very-far-reap-benefits-running
http://www.health.harvard.edu/blog/running-health-even-little-bit-good-little-probably-better-201407307310
http://www.medicaldaily.com/run-your-life-6-health-benefits-running-just-5-minutes-every-day-322050